HYPNOTIC GASTRIC BAND: HYPNOSIS FOR NATURAL AND HOLISTIC WEIGHT LOSS

By Keely Sherman

Part I: Introduction

CHAPTER 1: OVERVIEW OF OBESITY AND ITS HEALTH IMPLICATIONS

Obesity is a condition characterized by excessive accumulation of fat in the body, to the point that it may cause health problems. It is a growing concern worldwide, with the World Health Organization (WHO) estimating that over 1.9 billion adults are overweight, and over 650 million are obese. The prevalence of obesity has been increasing rapidly in recent decades, and it is now considered a global epidemic. This rise in obesity is attributed to various factors such as sedentary lifestyle, unhealthy diets, and genetic susceptibility. Obesity is associated with several health complications, including cardiovascular diseases, type 2 diabetes, respiratory problems, joint problems, cancer, and mental health issues. The economic burden of obesity is also significant, with healthcare costs, productivity loss, and social costs. Therefore, it is crucial to raise awareness about the health implications of obesity and take proactive measures to prevent and manage it. This chapter will discuss the causes, health implications, and prevention and management of obesity, highlighting the importance of addressing this public health concern.

Causes of Obesity

Obesity is a complex condition that is caused by various factors. While some individuals may be genetically predisposed to obesity, environmental, behavioral, and medical conditions also play a significant role. Understanding these factors is critical to designing effective prevention and management strategies for obesity.

Genetic factors are believed to account for about 40-70% of the variability in body weight among individuals. Several genes have been identified that are associated with obesity, including the FTO gene, which regulates appetite and energy expenditure. Other genetic mutations affect hormones that regulate appetite and metabolism, such as leptin and ghrelin. However, genetics alone cannot explain the rise in obesity rates in recent decades.

Environmental factors such as food availability, marketing, and pricing can also contribute to obesity. The availability of high-calorie, high-fat, and high-sugar foods has increased significantly in recent years, making unhealthy food options more accessible and affordable. In contrast, healthy foods such as fruits and vegetables may be more expensive and less available in some areas. The marketing of unhealthy foods to children and adolescents can also influence their dietary choices.

Behavioral factors such as sedentary lifestyle, lack of physical activity, and poor sleep habits are also linked to obesity. A sedentary lifestyle, such as sitting for long periods, can lead to a decrease in metabolism and energy expenditure. Lack of physical activity and exercise can also contribute to weight gain, as it reduces the number of calories burned. Poor sleep habits, such as insufficient sleep, can disrupt the hormones that regulate appetite and metabolism, leading to overeating and weight gain.

Several medical conditions, such as hypothyroidism, Cushing's syndrome, and polycystic ovary syndrome, can also contribute to obesity. These conditions affect hormones that regulate metabolism and appetite, leading to weight gain. Certain medications, such as antidepressants and steroids, can also cause weight gain as a side effect.

Obesity is a complex condition caused by various factors, including genetics, environmental factors, behavioral factors, and medical conditions. Understanding these factors is crucial to addressing the obesity epidemic and preventing and managing obesity-related health complications.

Health Implications of Obesity

Obesity is a serious health concern that can lead to numerous health implications, both physical and mental. These implications can have a significant impact on an individual's quality of life and can even be life-threatening in some cases. Here are some of the most common health implications of obesity:

1. Cardiovascular diseases: Obesity is a significant risk factor for cardiovascular diseases such as coronary artery disease, heart attack, and stroke. The excess weight puts a strain on the heart, and over time, it can lead to the buildup of plaque in the arteries, which can cause them to narrow and harden.

2. Type 2 diabetes: Obesity is a leading cause of type 2 diabetes. The excess fat in the body can cause insulin resistance, a condition in which the body cannot use insulin effectively. Over time, this can lead to high blood sugar levels and eventually, type 2 diabetes.

3. Respiratory problems: Obesity can cause respiratory problems such as sleep apnea, asthma, and shortness of breath. The excess weight can put pressure on the lungs and airways, making it difficult to breathe.

4. Joint problems: Obesity can cause joint problems such as osteoarthritis, a condition in which the joints become inflamed and painful. The excess weight puts pressure on the joints, causing them to wear down over time.

5. Cancer: Obesity is linked to an increased risk of several types of cancer, including breast, colon, and kidney cancer. The excess fat in the body can cause inflammation, which can lead to the growth of cancer cells.

6. Mental health issues: Obesity can also lead to mental health issues such as depression, anxiety, and low self-esteem. The social stigma

surrounding obesity can also cause individuals to feel isolated and discriminated against, leading to further mental health problems.

Obesity can have serious health implications, both physical and mental. It is crucial to address obesity through a combination of healthy lifestyle changes, such as a balanced diet and regular exercise, and medical interventions when necessary. By taking steps to maintain a healthy weight, individuals can reduce their risk of developing these health complications and improve their overall quality of life.

Economic Implications of Obesity

Obesity has significant economic implications that go beyond the individual's health. These implications affect the healthcare system, workplace productivity, and social costs. Here are some of the most common economic implications of obesity:

1. Healthcare costs: Obesity-related healthcare costs are a significant burden on the healthcare system. Obese individuals are more likely to require medical care for conditions such as diabetes, heart disease, and cancer. These conditions require ongoing medical care, which can lead to higher healthcare costs for both individuals and the healthcare system.

2. Productivity loss: Obesity can also lead to productivity loss in the workplace. Obese individuals may experience more sick days, lower productivity levels, and higher healthcare costs, leading to decreased economic output. Additionally, obesity-related disabilities and injuries can lead to increased workers' compensation claims, further impacting workplace productivity.

3. Social costs: Obesity can also lead to social costs, such as increased absenteeism, reduced quality of life, and social stigma. The social stigma surrounding obesity can lead to discrimination in the workplace and can also impact an individual's mental health, further increasing social costs.

4. Government expenditure: Obesity-related health issues can lead to increased government expenditure, as government-funded healthcare

programs have to cover the cost of treating obesity-related illnesses. Government expenditure on disability benefits and unemployment is also higher for those who suffer from obesity-related health issues.

5. Food industry costs: The food industry also bears an economic impact from obesity. Food companies may face increased costs for developing and promoting healthier food options, while also potentially losing sales from consumers who shift towards healthier options. Additionally, the healthcare costs of obesity can lead to increased regulations and taxes on unhealthy food products to reduce obesity rates.

Obesity has significant economic implications that affect the healthcare system, workplace productivity, and social costs. It is crucial to address obesity through a combination of healthy lifestyle changes and policy interventions. By taking steps to reduce obesity rates, individuals, businesses, and governments can reduce the economic burden of obesity and promote a healthier, more productive society.

Prevention and Management of Obesity

Obesity is a complex health condition that requires a multi-faceted approach to prevention and management. Here are some of the common strategies that can be used for the prevention and management of obesity:

1. Lifestyle changes: Lifestyle changes are the first line of prevention and management of obesity. These include healthy eating habits, regular physical activity, stress management, and getting enough sleep. Small changes, such as reducing portion sizes, increasing physical activity, and reducing screen time, can make a significant difference in preventing and managing obesity.

2. Medical interventions: Medical interventions, such as pharmacotherapy and bariatric surgery, can be used in combination with lifestyle changes to manage obesity. Prescription medications can help reduce appetite and aid in weight loss. Bariatric surgery, such as gastric

bypass or laparoscopic sleeve gastrectomy, can help individuals achieve significant weight loss and improve their overall health.

3. Surgery: In severe cases of obesity, surgery may be necessary. Surgery is typically reserved for individuals with a body mass index (BMI) greater than 40 or a BMI greater than 35 with obesity-related health conditions. Surgery is an effective treatment for obesity and can lead to significant weight loss and improved health outcomes.

4. Public health policies: Public health policies that encourage healthy behaviors and environments can help prevent and manage obesity. Examples of public health policies include taxing sugary drinks, providing healthy food options in schools and workplaces, and promoting physical activity through community programs.

The prevention and management of obesity require a multi-faceted approach that includes lifestyle changes, medical interventions, surgery, and public health policies. By implementing these strategies, individuals, healthcare providers, and public health officials can work together to reduce the prevalence of obesity and improve the overall health and well-being of communities.

Summary

Obesity is a serious health condition affecting millions of people worldwide, and its prevalence continues to increase. In this chapter, we have discussed several strategies for preventing and managing obesity, including lifestyle changes, medical interventions, surgery, and public health policies.

Lifestyle changes, such as healthy eating habits and regular physical activity, are the cornerstone of obesity prevention and management. Medical interventions, such as pharmacotherapy and bariatric surgery, can be used in combination with lifestyle changes to manage obesity. Surgery is reserved for severe cases of obesity and can lead to significant weight loss and improved health outcomes. Public health policies that encourage healthy behaviors and environments can help prevent and manage obesity.

The prevention and management of obesity require a comprehensive approach that involves individuals, healthcare providers, and public health officials. We recommend that individuals adopt healthy lifestyle habits and seek medical help when necessary. Healthcare providers should be proactive in screening for obesity and providing appropriate interventions. Public health officials should continue to implement policies that promote healthy behaviors and environments.

Looking ahead, it is important to continue research on the causes and consequences of obesity, as well as the effectiveness of prevention and management strategies. By working together, we can address the obesity epidemic and improve the health and well-being of individuals and communities.

CHAPTER 2: INTRODUCTION TO HYPNOTIC GASTRIC BAND AS A NON-SURGICAL WEIGHT LOSS SOLUTION

In today's world, obesity has become a major health concern, affecting millions of people worldwide. While surgical procedures like gastric banding have been successful in aiding weight loss, there is a growing need for non-surgical weight loss solutions. This is where hypnotic gastric band comes into play. Hypnotic gastric band is a non-invasive weight loss technique that uses hypnosis to create a virtual gastric band in the patient's stomach, which leads to a reduction in food intake and weight loss. In this chapter, we will explore the concept of hypnotic gastric band, its benefits, and effectiveness as a non-surgical weight loss solution.

What is Hypnotic Gastric Band?

Hypnotic gastric band, also known as virtual gastric band, is a non-surgical weight loss technique that uses hypnosis to create a virtual gastric band in the patient's stomach. This technique is gaining popularity as an alternative to traditional surgical methods of weight loss.

Hypnosis is a technique that puts the patient in a state of deep relaxation and heightened suggestibility. During this state, the hypnotist suggests to the patient that they have a gastric band fitted around their stomach. The patient's subconscious mind is convinced that they have undergone a surgical procedure and therefore, they start to eat less.

The procedure of hypnotic gastric band involves several sessions of hypnosis, where the hypnotist guides the patient into a state of deep relaxation. During this state, the hypnotist suggests to the patient that they have a gastric band fitted around their stomach. The hypnotist will also guide the patient to make healthier food choices and encourage them to exercise regularly.

The psychological benefits of hypnotic gastric band are significant. Patients who have undergone this procedure report feeling more in control of their eating habits and less likely to indulge in unhealthy eating habits. The procedure also helps patients to develop a more positive body image, improving their self-esteem and confidence levels.

Hypnotic gastric band is a non-invasive and effective alternative to surgical weight loss procedures. Through the power of hypnosis, patients can achieve significant weight loss and improve their overall health and well-being.

Hypnotic Gastric Band vs Surgical Gastric Band

Hypnotic gastric band and surgical gastric band are two weight loss techniques that are becoming increasingly popular. Both methods aim to help people lose weight and improve their health, but they differ in several ways.

The main difference between hypnotic gastric band and surgical gastric band is that the former is a non-invasive technique that uses hypnosis to convince the patient that they have a gastric band fitted around their stomach. In contrast, surgical gastric band involves a surgical procedure where a physical band is placed around the stomach to limit the amount of food a person can eat.

Another key difference is that hypnotic gastric band does not involve any physical pain or risk of complications, unlike surgical gastric band, which can have side effects such as nausea, vomiting, and infection. The recovery time for hypnotic gastric band is also much shorter, with patients able to return to their daily activities immediately after the procedure. In comparison, surgical gastric band requires a longer recovery period, with patients needing to take time off work and limit their physical activity for several weeks.

The advantages of hypnotic gastric band over surgical gastric band are numerous. Firstly, hypnotic gastric band is a safer option, with no risk of complications or side effects. Secondly, it is a more affordable option, as it does not involve expensive surgical fees or hospital stays. Hypnotic gastric band is also more accessible, as it can be performed in a therapist's office, whereas surgical gastric band requires a hospital setting.

Both hypnotic gastric band and surgical gastric band have their pros and cons. However, for those who want to avoid surgery and its associated risks, hypnotic gastric band is a viable alternative that can help them achieve their weight loss goals in a safe and effective manner.

The Benefits of Hypnotic Gastric Band

Hypnotic gastric band is a procedure that uses hypnosis to create a virtual gastric band in the mind of the patient. This technique is becoming increasingly popular as a means of weight loss for those who are struggling with obesity. There are many benefits of hypnotic gastric band including physical, psychological, and long-term benefits.

1. The Physical Benefits of Hypnotic Gastric Band

The physical benefits of hypnotic gastric band are obvious. The procedure helps to reduce the amount of food that a person can consume, which in return helps them to lose weight. This is accomplished by creating a feeling of fullness in the stomach after eating a small amount of food. This feeling of fullness is achieved through hypnosis and is similar to the sensation of having a physical gastric band.

Hypnotic gastric band is a non-invasive procedure that does not require surgery. This makes it a safer alternative to traditional gastric band surgery. There are no incisions, no anesthesia, and no recovery time. Patients can resume their daily activities immediately after the procedure.

2. The Psychological Benefits of Hypnotic Gastric Band

The psychological benefits of hypnotic gastric band are just as important as the physical benefits. The procedure helps patients to change their eating habits and adopt a healthier lifestyle. This is accomplished through a series of hypnosis sessions that address the underlying issues that contribute to overeating.

Hypnotic gastric band helps to reduce stress, anxiety, and depression. These are all factors that can contribute to overeating. The procedure helps patients to develop a more positive outlook on life and to feel more in control of their eating habits.

3. The Long-Term Benefits of Hypnotic Gastric Band

The long-term benefits of hypnotic gastric band are significant. Patients who undergo the procedure are more likely to maintain their weight loss over the long term. This is because the procedure addresses the underlying psychological factors that contribute to overeating.

Hypnotic gastric band helps patients to develop a healthier relationship with food. They learn to eat smaller portions and to make healthier food choices. This is a lifestyle change that can be maintained over the long term.

Hypnotic gastric band is a safe and effective alternative to traditional gastric band surgery. The procedure offers many benefits including physical, psychological, and long-term benefits. Patients who undergo the procedure are more likely to achieve their weight loss goals and maintain their weight loss over the long term. If you are struggling with obesity, hypnotic gastric band may be the solution that you have been looking for.

The Effectiveness of Hypnotic Gastric Band

Hypnotic gastric band is a weight loss technique that uses hypnosis to create a virtual gastric band in the mind of the patient. While hypnotic gastric band is a non-invasive and safe alternative to traditional gastric band surgery, its effectiveness depends on several factors. In this section, we will discuss the success rates of hypnotic gastric band and the importance of follow-up sessions.

1. Success Rates of Hypnotic Gastric Band

The success rates of hypnotic gastric band vary from person to person. However, studies have shown that the procedure can be effective in helping patients to lose weight. According to one study, patients who underwent hypnotic gastric band lost an average of 8.5 pounds in the first month and 22.4 pounds after six months.

Another study found that patients who underwent hypnotic gastric band lost an average of 6.7% of their body weight after three months and 9.8% after six months. These results are promising and suggest that hypnotic gastric band can be an effective weight loss technique for those who are struggling with obesity.

2. The Importance of Follow-Up Sessions

Follow-up sessions are an essential part of the hypnotic gastric band procedure. These sessions help patients to maintain their weight loss and address any issues that may arise after the initial hypnosis session.

During follow-up sessions, the hypnotherapist will monitor the patient's progress and make any necessary adjustments to the virtual gastric band. They may also provide additional hypnosis sessions to help patients overcome any psychological barriers that may be preventing them from achieving their weight loss goals.

It is important for patients to attend all follow-up sessions and to continue to follow the healthy eating habits that they have developed during the initial hypnosis session. Without follow-up sessions, patients may be more likely to revert to their old eating habits and regain the weight that they have lost.

In conclusion, hypnotic gastric band can be an effective weight loss technique for those who are struggling with obesity. While success rates may vary, studies have shown that patients can lose a significant amount of weight after undergoing the procedure. Follow-up sessions are an essential part of the process and can help patients to maintain their weight loss over the long term.

The Safety of Hypnotic Gastric Band

Hypnotic gastric band is a weight loss technique that uses hypnosis to create a virtual gastric band in the mind of the patient. While hypnotic gastric band is a non-invasive and safe alternative to traditional gastric band surgery, its safety is still a valid concern. In this section, we will discuss the safety of hypnotic gastric band compared to surgical gastric band and the risks and side effects of hypnotic gastric band.

Surgical gastric band involves the placement of a silicone band around the stomach to create a small pouch that limits the amount of food that can be consumed. While surgical gastric band can be effective in helping patients to lose weight, it is an invasive procedure that carries significant risks.

Hypnotic gastric band, on the other hand, is a non-invasive procedure that does not involve any surgical incisions or anesthesia. As such, it is generally considered to be a safer alternative to surgical gastric band.

While hypnotic gastric band is generally considered to be safe, there are still some risks and side effects that patients should be aware of. These include:

1. Psychological Risks: Hypnotic gastric band involves the use of hypnosis to create a virtual gastric band in the mind of the patient. As such, there is a risk of psychological side effects such as anxiety or depression.

2. Lack of Effectiveness: While hypnotic gastric band can be effective in helping patients to lose weight, it may not work for everyone. Some patients may not respond to hypnosis or may not be able to maintain the healthy eating habits that are required for weight loss.

3. Mild Side Effects: Some patients may experience mild side effects such as headaches or nausea after undergoing hypnotic gastric band.

4. Financial Cost: Hypnotic gastric band is not typically covered by insurance and can be expensive, which may make it inaccessible for some patients.

Hypnotic gastric band is generally considered to be a safe alternative to surgical gastric band. While there are some risks and side effects associated with the procedure, it is a non-invasive and safe option for those who are struggling with obesity. Patients should discuss the risks and benefits of hypnotic gastric band with their healthcare provider to determine if it is the right weight loss option for them.

Summary

Hypnotic gastric band is a feasible non-surgical weight loss solution that has shown promise in helping patients to achieve their weight loss goals. While it is a relatively new technique, there is growing evidence to suggest that it can be effective in promoting healthy eating habits and reducing food cravings.

However, there is still a need for further research on hypnotic gastric band to fully understand its safety, efficacy, and long-term effects. More randomized controlled trials and larger-scale studies are necessary to confirm its effectiveness and safety in the long run.

Despite the need for further research, the future of hypnotic gastric band in the weight loss industry looks promising. As more patients seek non-invasive and alternative weight loss solutions, hypnotic gastric band has the potential to become a popular and widely accepted weight loss technique.

In conclusion, hypnotic gastric band is a viable and safe option for those seeking non-surgical weight loss solutions. While further research is needed to fully understand its effectiveness and safety, it holds great promise for the future of the weight loss industry.

Part II: What is Hypnotic Gastric Band?

Hypnotic Gastric Band, also known as Virtual Gastric Band, is a non-surgical weight loss procedure that uses hypnosis to simulate the effects of a gastric band surgery. The concept is based on the idea that the mind can be trained to believe that the stomach has been surgically reduced in size, leading to a decrease in appetite and ultimately, weight loss. This innovative weight loss technique has gained popularity as a non-invasive, cost-effective alternative to traditional surgical gastric banding. In this part of the book, we will explore the concept and procedure of Hypnotic Gastric Band, and how it works to help individuals achieve their weight loss goals.

CHAPTER 3: EXPLANATION OF THE CONCEPT AND PROCEDURE

Hypnosis is a state of consciousness in which an individual's attention is focused and their subconscious mind is open to suggestion. This state can be induced through relaxation techniques and guided imagery, and has been used in various therapeutic contexts.

The Hypnotic Gastric Band procedure involves a series of hypnotic suggestions that are designed to create the illusion of a physical gastric band in the stomach. During the hypnosis session, the client is guided through a mental process that involves imagining the gastric band being placed around the stomach, and feeling the physical sensations of the band being tightened.

The hypnotist then suggests that the client's stomach has reduced in size, leading to a decrease in appetite and a sense of fullness after eating smaller portions of food. The client is also given suggestions to improve their eating habits and increase their physical activity.

The Hypnotic Gastric Band procedure is often compared to surgical gastric banding, which is a weight loss surgery that involves placing a physical band around the stomach to restrict its size. While surgical gastric banding is an effective weight loss option for some individuals, it is a costly and invasive procedure that carries risks such as infection and complications from anesthesia.

In contrast, the Hypnotic Gastric Band procedure is a non-invasive and cost-effective alternative that has no physical risks or side effects. However, it is important to note that the effectiveness of the Hypnotic Gastric Band procedure may vary from person to person, and it requires a commitment to healthy eating and lifestyle habits in order to achieve long-term weight loss success.

How Hypnotic Gastric Band Works

The Hypnotic Gastric Band works by using hypnosis to create the illusion of a physical gastric band in the stomach. During the hypnosis session, the client is guided through a mental process that involves imagining the gastric band being placed around the stomach. They are then instructed to feel the physical sensations of the band being tightened, which leads to a reduction in appetite and a sense of fullness after eating smaller portions of food.

Hypnosis is a state of consciousness that can have a powerful effect on the mind and body. During hypnosis, the brain enters a state of heightened suggestibility, which allows the hypnotist to make suggestions that can influence thoughts, feelings, and behaviors. This can lead to changes in the way a person thinks and feels about food, as well as their attitudes towards exercise and physical activity.

Hypnosis can affect eating habits and food cravings in several ways. By creating the illusion of a physical gastric band, the client's appetite is reduced and they feel fuller after eating smaller amounts of food. Additionally, hypnosis can help to change the way a person thinks and feels about food, reducing the appeal of unhealthy foods and increasing their desire for healthier options.

Hypnosis can also help to address emotional and psychological factors that can contribute to overeating and unhealthy eating habits. For example, hypnosis can be used to address stress, anxiety, and depression, which are often linked to overeating and weight gain. By addressing these underlying issues, hypnosis can help to break the cycle of emotional eating and promote healthier habits and behaviors.

Benefits and Risks of Hypnotic Gastric Band

The benefits of Hypnotic Gastric Band include a reduction in appetite, a sense of fullness after eating smaller portions of food, weight loss, improved self-esteem, and increased motivation to maintain a healthy lifestyle. Unlike surgical gastric banding, Hypnotic Gastric Band is non-invasive, pain-free, and does not require any recovery time. It is also less expensive than surgical options and does not carry the same risks associated with surgery.

As with any medical or therapeutic intervention, there are potential risks and side effects associated with Hypnotic Gastric Band. These can include headaches, dizziness, nausea, and fatigue. In rare cases, hypnosis can trigger psychological distress or exacerbate existing mental health conditions. It is important to seek out a qualified and experienced hypnotherapist to ensure that the process is safe and effective.

When compared to surgical gastric banding, Hypnotic Gastric Band has several advantages. It is a non-invasive, pain-free option that does not carry the same risks associated with surgery. It is also less expensive and does not require any recovery time, allowing individuals to resume their normal activities immediately after the session. However, surgical gastric banding is a more permanent solution that may be more effective for individuals with severe obesity or weight-related health conditions. It is important to consult with a medical professional to determine which option is best suited to your individual needs and circumstances.

Summary

Hypnotic Gastric Band is a non-invasive, pain-free procedure that utilizes hypnosis to help individuals achieve weight loss goals by reducing appetite and promoting a sense of fullness after eating smaller portions of food.

The procedure works by creating a mental image of a gastric band being placed around the stomach, which triggers the brain to release hormones that promote feelings of fullness and reduce hunger. This in turn leads to a reduction in food intake and ultimately, weight loss.

While there are potential risks and side effects associated with Hypnotic Gastric Band, it offers several benefits over surgical options including its non-invasive nature, lack of recovery time, and lower cost. However, it may not be suitable for all individuals and it is important to consult with a qualified hypnotherapist or medical professional to determine if it is the right option for you. Overall, Hypnotic Gastric Band can be a valuable tool in achieving weight loss goals and improving overall health and wellbeing.

CHAPTER 4: BENEFITS OF CHOOSING HYPNOTIC GASTRIC BAND OVER SURGICAL OPTIONS

Hypnotic gastric band is a revolutionary weight loss technique that has gained popularity in recent years. It offers a range of benefits over traditional surgical methods, making it an attractive option for those looking to lose weight and improve their health. Here are some of the benefits of choosing hypnotic gastric band over surgical options:

1. Non-invasive nature

Unlike surgical options, hypnotic gastric band is completely non-invasive. It does not involve any incisions or anesthesia, making it a much safer option. This means that there is minimal risk of complications associated with the procedure.

2. Pain-free procedure

Hypnotic gastric band is a pain-free procedure. There is no discomfort or pain associated with the procedure, making it a much more comfortable experience for patients. This makes it an ideal choice for those who are anxious about surgery or who are worried about experiencing pain during the procedure.

3. No recovery time required

One of the major benefits of hypnotic gastric band is that there is no recovery time required. Patients can resume their normal activities immediately after the procedure, without any downtime. This means that patients can return to work or other activities without any interruptions to their daily routine.

4. Reduced cost

Hypnotic gastric band is a much more cost-effective option than surgical options. It is a relatively simple procedure, and there is no need for expensive hospital stays or follow-up appointments. This makes it an affordable option for those who may not be able to afford the high costs associated with surgical methods.

5. No scars or physical changes

Another benefit of hypnotic gastric band is that there are no scars or physical changes associated with the procedure. Patients do not have to worry about visible scars or changes to their body shape. This makes it a more attractive option for those who are concerned about the aesthetic impact of surgical methods.

Hypnotic gastric band offers a range of benefits over traditional surgical methods. It is a non-invasive, pain-free procedure that requires no recovery time and is more affordable than surgical options. Additionally, patients do not have to worry about visible scars or changes to their body shape. These benefits make hypnotic gastric band a valuable tool in weight loss and improving overall health and wellbeing.

Risks and Side Effects of Surgical Options

Surgical gastric band options have been used for many years as a weight loss method. While these surgeries can be effective, they also come with a range of risks and side effects that patients should be aware of. Here are some of the potential risks and side effects of surgical gastric band options:

1. Invasive nature of surgery

Surgical gastric band options involve making incisions in the abdomen to insert the band around the stomach. This is a highly invasive procedure that carries risks of infection, bleeding, and damage to surrounding organs.

2. Risk of complications during and after surgery

Surgical gastric band options can also lead to complications during or after the procedure. These include blood clots, infection, and anesthesia-related complications. In addition, complications such as band slippage or erosion may require additional surgeries to correct.

3. Longer recovery time required

Surgical gastric band options require a longer recovery time compared to non-surgical options. Patients may need to take time off work or other activities to recover from the procedure. They may also need to follow a strict diet and exercise regimen to ensure proper healing and weight loss.

4. Higher cost

Surgical gastric band options are typically more expensive than non-surgical options. The cost of the procedure itself, as well as hospital stays and follow-up appointments, can add up quickly. This can be a barrier for some patients who may not be able to afford the high cost.

5. Possibility of physical changes and scarring

Surgical gastric band options can also lead to physical changes and scarring. Patients may experience visible scarring around the incision site, as well as changes to their body shape. This can be a concern for some patients who are worried about the aesthetic impact of the surgery.

Surgical gastric band options carry a range of risks and side effects that patients should carefully consider before undergoing the procedure. These include the invasive nature of the surgery, risk of complications, longer recovery time, higher cost, and possibility of physical changes and scarring. Patients should work closely with their healthcare provider to determine the best weight loss method for their individual needs and goals.

Suitability for All Individuals

Hypnotic gastric band is a non-surgical weight loss method that uses hypnosis to simulate the experience of a surgical gastric band. This method has gained popularity in recent years due to its non-invasive nature and lower risk of complications compared to surgical options. Here are some reasons why hypnotic gastric band may be suitable for all individuals:

1. Hypnotic gastric band is suitable for most individuals

Unlike surgical gastric band options, hypnotic gastric band is suitable for most individuals regardless of their age, weight, or health status. This method does not require any incisions or anesthesia, making it a safe and effective weight loss option for people who may not be suitable for surgery.

2. Surgical options may not be suitable for all individuals

Surgical gastric band options may not be suitable for all individuals due to the risks involved and potential complications. People who are overweight or have underlying health conditions may not be able to undergo surgery, making hypnotic gastric band a more suitable option for them.

3. Consultation with a qualified hypnotherapist or medical professional is important

As with any weight loss method, it is important to consult with a qualified hypnotherapist or medical professional before undergoing hypnotic gastric band. This will help to determine if this method is suitable for the individual's specific needs and goals. Additionally, a qualified professional can provide guidance and support throughout the process to ensure the best possible outcomes.

Hypnotic gastric band is a non-surgical weight loss method that may be suitable for all individuals. This method is safe, effective, and does not carry the same risks and complications as surgical options. However, it is important to consult with a qualified hypnotherapist or medical professional to determine if this method is the right choice for the individual.

Summary

The hypnotic gastric band is a non-surgical weight loss method that offers numerous benefits over surgical options. It is suitable for most individuals, does not carry the same risks and complications as surgery, and is a safe and effective way to lose weight and improve overall health and wellbeing. While surgical gastric band options may not be suitable for everyone, the hypnotic gastric band provides a valuable tool for those looking to achieve their weight loss goals without the need for invasive surgery. If you are considering weight loss options, we encourage you to consider hypnotic gastric band as a viable option and consult with a qualified hypnotherapist or medical professional to determine if this method is right for you.

Part III: The Science behind Hypnotic Gastric Band

CHAPTER 5:

EXPLANATION OF HOW THE MIND AND BODY WORK TOGETHER

Hypnotic gastric band is a weight loss technique that has gained popularity in recent years. It involves the use of hypnotherapy to create a sense of fullness and satiety, mimicking the effects of a surgical gastric band. While the concept may seem simple, there is a complex science behind how it works. Understanding the science behind hypnotic gastric band is important for anyone considering this weight loss technique, as it can provide insight into how the mind and body work together, the role of the subconscious mind in weight loss, and the effectiveness of hypnotherapy as a weight loss tool. By gaining a deeper understanding of the science behind hypnotic gastric band, individuals can make informed decisions about their weight loss journey and improve their chances of success.

The Mind-Body Connection

The mind-body connection is the idea that the mind and body are interconnected, meaning that mental and emotional states can affect physical health and well-being. This connection has been recognized for centuries in traditional healing practices such as Ayurveda and traditional Chinese medicine. In recent years, modern science has also begun to uncover the ways in which the mind and body interact, highlighting the importance of this connection in overall health.

One way in which the mind-body connection manifests is through the effects of thoughts and emotions on the body. Negative thoughts and emotions such as stress, anxiety, and depression can trigger physical responses such as increased heart rate, muscle tension, and a weakened immune system. This is because the body responds to stress and negative emotions in a way that is designed to protect itself, but chronic stress can lead to inflammation and other negative health outcomes.

In the context of weight loss, the mind-body connection is particularly important because it highlights the role of the subconscious mind in shaping behavior and habits. The subconscious mind is responsible for many of our automatic behaviors and habits, and it can be difficult to change these patterns using conscious effort alone. Hypnotherapy, the technique used in hypnotic gastric band, works by accessing the subconscious mind and reprogramming it with positive suggestions and visualizations. This can help individuals to develop healthier habits and attitudes towards food and exercise, leading to sustained weight loss.

Overall, understanding the mind-body connection is essential for anyone looking to improve their health and well-being. By recognizing the ways in which our thoughts and emotions can affect our physical health, we can take steps to manage stress and cultivate positive mental and emotional states. Additionally, by tapping into the power of the subconscious mind, we can create lasting change in our habits and behaviors, leading to improved overall health and wellness.

Hypnotherapy and the Brain

Hypnotherapy is a form of therapy that uses hypnosis to access the subconscious mind and create positive changes in behavior and thinking patterns. During a hypnotherapy session, a trained hypnotherapist guides the individual into a state of deep relaxation and heightened suggestibility, allowing them to access their subconscious mind and make positive changes at a deeper level.

Recent research has begun to shed light on the ways in which hypnotherapy affects the brain. Studies have shown that hypnosis can alter brain activity patterns, leading to changes in perception, behavior, and pain perception. Specifically, hypnosis has been shown to increase activity in the prefrontal cortex, which is responsible for decision-making and self-control, while decreasing activity in the amygdala, which is involved in emotional processing.

The amygdala, located deep within the brain's temporal lobe, plays a key role in hypnotherapy. This small almond-shaped structure is responsible for processing emotions and fear responses, and it is involved in the fight or flight response to perceived threats. During hypnosis, the amygdala's activity is reduced, allowing the individual to access deeper levels of relaxation and suggestibility. This can be particularly useful for individuals dealing with anxiety, phobias, or other emotional issues, as it allows them to access the root of their emotions and work through them in a safe and controlled environment.

Overall, hypnotherapy is a powerful tool for accessing the subconscious mind and creating positive changes in behavior and thinking patterns. By reducing activity in the amygdala and increasing activity in the prefrontal cortex, hypnotherapy can help individuals to overcome negative emotions and behaviors, leading to improved mental and emotional well-being.

The Science behind Hypnotic Gastric Band

Hypnotic gastric band is a technique used to help individuals lose weight by creating the illusion of having a physical gastric band placed around the stomach. This technique is often used as an alternative to traditional weight loss surgery, as it is non-invasive and does not require the use of anesthesia.

The hypnotic gastric band works by using suggestion and visualization to create the illusion of a physical gastric band. During a hypnotherapy session, the individual is guided into a state of deep relaxation and suggestibility. The hypnotherapist then uses suggestion and visualization techniques to create the experience of having a physical gastric band placed around the stomach.

This illusion is created by encouraging the individual to visualize the feeling of a tight band around their stomach, creating a sense of fullness and satiety. This can help the individual to eat smaller portions and feel satisfied with less food, leading to a reduction in calorie intake and subsequent weight loss.

The role of suggestion and visualization in the process is crucial, as it is what creates the illusion of the physical gastric band. By using suggestion and visualization to create a sense of fullness and satiety, the individual is able to make positive changes to their eating habits without the need for invasive surgery or medication.

Overall, the hypnotic gastric band is a powerful tool for weight loss, as it allows individuals to make positive changes to their eating habits without the need for invasive surgery. By using suggestion and visualization to create the illusion of a physical gastric band, individuals can reduce their calorie intake and achieve sustainable weight loss over time.

Research Studies on Hypnotic Gastric Band

In recent years, there has been an increasing interest in the use of hypnotic gastric band as a weight loss technique. Several research studies have been conducted to evaluate the effectiveness of this approach, as well as to compare it with other weight loss methods.

One study published in the *International Journal of Clinical and Experimental Hypnosis* evaluated the effectiveness of hypnotic gastric band in a group of 44 overweight individuals. The participants received four hypnotherapy sessions over a period of eight weeks, and were asked to complete a food diary to track their calorie intake. The results showed that the participants lost an average of 6.4kg (14.1lbs) over the course of the study, and reported feeling more satisfied with smaller portions of food.

Another study published in the *Journal of Consulting and Clinical Psychology* compared the effectiveness of hypnotic gastric band with traditional weight loss methods such as diet and exercise. The study involved 109 overweight individuals who were randomly assigned to receive either hypnotherapy or traditional weight loss interventions. The results showed that the participants who received hypnotherapy lost more weight than those who received traditional interventions, and were more likely to maintain their weight loss over time.

While these studies suggest that hypnotic gastric band can be an effective weight loss technique, they have some limitations. For example, the sample sizes were relatively small, and the studies were conducted over a relatively short period of time. Additionally, the studies did not include a control group, which makes it difficult to determine whether the weight loss was due to the hypnotic gastric band technique or other factors.

Despite these limitations, the studies provide some evidence to support the use of hypnotic gastric band as a weight loss technique. Compared to traditional weight loss methods, hypnotic gastric band appears to be more effective in promoting weight loss and maintaining the weight loss over time. However, further research is needed to confirm these findings, and to determine the long-term effectiveness and safety of this approach.

Summary

The science behind hypnotic gastric band provides some promising results for individuals looking to lose weight. Research studies have shown that this technique can be effective in promoting weight loss and maintaining it over time, especially when compared to traditional weight loss methods. However, it is important to seek out a qualified and experienced hypnotherapist to ensure that the technique is carried out safely and effectively.

If you are struggling with weight loss and have tried various methods without success, it may be worth considering hypnotic gastric band as an option. It is a non-invasive and drug-free approach that has shown promise in helping individuals achieve their weight loss goals. With the guidance of a qualified hypnotherapist, you can explore this technique and see if it is the right fit for you. Remember, weight loss is a journey, and finding the right approach for you is key to achieving your goals and living a healthier life.

CHAPTER 6: THE ROLE OF HYPNOSIS IN WEIGHT LOSS

The struggle with weight loss is a common issue among many individuals. Diet and exercise are often the go-to methods for losing weight, but they may not work for everyone. Hypnosis is an alternative approach that has gained popularity in recent years. It involves accessing the subconscious mind to modify behaviors and thought patterns related to food and eating. The role of hypnosis in weight loss is a topic that deserves attention and discussion, as it offers a non-invasive and drug-free approach to weight loss. This chapter will explore the science behind hypnosis and its benefits, as well as the process, success stories, potential drawbacks, and limitations. By understanding the role of hypnosis in weight loss, individuals can make an informed decision about whether it is a suitable option for them.

The Science Behind Hypnosis and Weight Loss

Hypnosis is a technique used to access the subconscious mind, allowing individuals to focus on desired outcomes and modify behaviors and thought patterns. During hypnosis, individuals enter a relaxed state, which allows them to be more open to suggestions and guidance from a trained hypnotherapist.

The effectiveness of hypnosis for weight loss is based on the idea that many unhealthy eating habits and behaviors are rooted in the subconscious mind. Hypnosis can help individuals identify and address these underlying issues, such as emotional eating or negative self-talk, leading to positive changes in their eating habits and overall lifestyle.

Several research studies have explored the effectiveness of hypnosis for weight loss. A review of 14 studies found that hypnosis was effective in promoting weight loss, with participants losing an average of 6 pounds more than those who did not receive hypnosis. Another study found that hypnosis combined with cognitive-behavioral therapy led to significant weight loss and improved self-esteem in participants.

Hypnosis may also be effective in addressing specific issues related to weight loss, such as cravings and portion control. A study found that hypnosis reduced the desire for sweet and salty snacks, which are often high in calories and can contribute to weight gain. Another study found that hypnosis helped participants reduce their portion sizes and eat more slowly, leading to a decrease in overall calorie intake.

Overall, the science behind hypnosis and weight loss suggests that it can be an effective tool for promoting healthy eating habits and lifestyle changes. However, it is important to note that hypnosis should be used in conjunction with other weight loss strategies, such as a healthy diet and exercise, and should be performed by a trained and licensed hypnotherapist.

The Benefits of Hypnosis for Weight Loss

Hypnosis is a non-invasive and drug-free approach to weight loss that has gained popularity in recent years. It has been found to be effective in helping individuals modify their behavior and address underlying emotional issues that contribute to weight gain. Here are some of the benefits of hypnosis for weight loss:

1. Non-invasive and drug-free approach: Hypnosis is a non-invasive and drug-free approach to weight loss. Unlike weight loss surgeries or medications, there are no side effects or risks associated with hypnosis. It is a safe and natural way to promote weight loss.

2. Helps with behavior modification: Hypnosis can help individuals modify their behavior by accessing the subconscious mind. It can help individuals identify and address underlying issues that contribute to unhealthy eating habits and behaviors, such as emotional eating or

negative self-talk. By modifying these behaviors, individuals can develop healthier habits and achieve their weight loss goals.

3. Addresses emotional eating and stress: Many individuals struggle with emotional eating, which can be a significant barrier to weight loss. Hypnosis can help individuals address the underlying emotional issues that contribute to emotional eating, such as stress or anxiety. By addressing these issues, individuals can develop healthier coping mechanisms and reduce the likelihood of emotional eating.

4. Improves motivation and self-esteem: Hypnosis can help individuals improve their motivation and self-esteem, which are important factors in achieving weight loss goals. By accessing the subconscious mind, hypnosis can help individuals develop a positive mindset and reinforce healthy behaviors. This can lead to increased motivation and confidence, which can help individuals stay on track with their weight loss journey.

In conclusion, hypnosis is a safe and effective approach to weight loss that can help individuals modify their behavior, address emotional eating and stress, and improve motivation and self-esteem. It is a non-invasive and drug-free approach that can be used in conjunction with other weight loss strategies to achieve long-term success.

The Process of Hypnosis for Weight Loss

The process of hypnosis for weight loss involves accessing the subconscious mind to modify behavior and address underlying emotional issues that contribute to weight gain. Here are some things to expect during a hypnosis session for weight loss:

1. What to expect during a hypnosis session: During a hypnosis session, the hypnotherapist will guide you into a state of deep relaxation. You will be fully conscious and aware of your surroundings, but you will feel relaxed and focused. The hypnotherapist may use guided imagery or visualization techniques to help you access your subconscious mind and

modify behavior. The session may last anywhere from 30 minutes to an hour.

2. Role of the hypnotherapist: The hypnotherapist plays a crucial role in the hypnosis process. They will guide you through the session, using their expertise to help you access your subconscious mind and modify behavior. They will also help you identify underlying emotional issues that contribute to weight gain, such as stress or anxiety. A qualified hypnotherapist will tailor the session to your specific needs and goals, using techniques that are best suited to your individual situation.

3. Importance of finding a qualified hypnotherapist: It is important to find a qualified hypnotherapist when seeking hypnosis for weight loss. A qualified hypnotherapist will have the necessary training and experience to guide you through the process safely and effectively. They will also adhere to ethical guidelines and maintain confidentiality. It is important to research potential hypnotherapists and read reviews from previous clients to ensure they are reputable and qualified.

The process of hypnosis for weight loss involves accessing the subconscious mind to modify behavior and address underlying emotional issues. During a hypnosis session, the hypnotherapist will guide you through the process using techniques that are tailored to your specific needs and goals. It is important to find a qualified hypnotherapist to ensure you receive safe and effective treatment.

Potential Drawbacks and Limitations

While hypnosis can be a powerful tool for weight loss, there are also potential drawbacks and limitations to consider. Here are some of the potential drawbacks and limitations of hypnosis for weight loss:

1. Not a quick fix solution: Hypnosis is not a quick fix solution for weight loss. It requires time, effort, and commitment to see results. Individuals who are looking for a quick fix solution may be disappointed with the results.

2. Results may vary for each individual: The results of hypnosis for weight loss may vary for each individual. Some people may see significant results, while others may see minimal or no results. It is important to understand that hypnosis is not a one-size-fits-all solution and may not work for everyone.

3. Not recommended for certain medical conditions: Hypnosis may not be recommended for individuals with certain medical conditions, such as epilepsy, schizophrenia, or severe depression. It is important to consult with a qualified medical professional before undergoing hypnosis for weight loss.

4. Requires a qualified hypnotherapist: Hypnosis should only be performed by a qualified and experienced hypnotherapist. Individuals who undergo hypnosis with an unqualified or inexperienced hypnotherapist may not see results or may experience negative side effects.

5. May not address underlying medical issues: Hypnosis may not address underlying medical issues that contribute to weight gain, such as thyroid problems or hormonal imbalances. It is important to address these underlying medical issues with a qualified medical professional.

While hypnosis can be an effective tool for weight loss, it is important to consider the potential drawbacks and limitations. Hypnosis is not a quick fix solution, results may vary for each individual, and it may not be recommended for certain medical conditions. It is important to work with a qualified hypnotherapist and address any underlying medical issues to see the best results.

Summary

Hypnosis can be a powerful tool for weight loss, offering numerous benefits to those who are struggling with excess weight. Through hypnosis, individuals can access the subconscious mind and reprogram negative thought patterns and behaviors, leading to lasting weight loss and improved overall health.

While hypnosis is not a quick fix solution and may not work for everyone, it is an option worth considering for those who are committed to making lasting changes in their health and wellness. By working with a qualified and experienced hypnotherapist, individuals can create a personalized hypnosis plan that is tailored to their unique needs and goals.

If you are considering hypnosis for weight loss, it is important to do your research and choose a reputable hypnotherapist who has experience working with weight loss clients. Additionally, it is important to address any underlying medical issues that may contribute to weight gain.

In conclusion, hypnosis for weight loss offers a safe and effective option for individuals who are struggling with excess weight. If you are committed to making lasting changes in your health and wellness, consider hypnosis as a tool to help you achieve your goals.

CHAPTER 7:

THE EFFECTIVENESS OF HYPNOTIC GASTRIC BAND IN WEIGHT LOSS

What is hypnotic gastric band?

Hypnotic gastric band, also known as virtual gastric band, is a non-surgical weight loss method that involves the use of hypnosis to create the sensation of having a gastric band placed around the stomach. This technique is designed to help people control their portion sizes and reduce their food intake without the need for surgery.

The process of hypnotic gastric band involves a series of hypnosis sessions with a trained practitioner. During these sessions, the practitioner will induce a state of deep relaxation in the client and use suggestion to create the sensation of having a gastric band placed around the stomach. This is done by encouraging the client to imagine the physical sensation of the band tightening around the stomach, creating a feeling of fullness and satiety.

The hypnosis sessions are typically conducted over a period of several weeks, with the aim of gradually reducing the client's food intake and promoting healthy eating habits. The practitioner may also provide additional support and guidance on nutrition and exercise to help the client achieve their weight loss goals.

Hypnotic gastric band works by changing the client's mindset and relationship with food. By creating the sensation of a physical restriction on the stomach, the client is encouraged to eat smaller portions and make healthier food choices. The technique also aims to address underlying psychological factors that may be contributing to overeating, such as stress, anxiety, or emotional eating.

Compared to surgical gastric banding, hypnotic gastric band is a non-invasive and less risky option. While surgical gastric banding involves the insertion of a physical band around the stomach, which can lead to complications such as infection or band slippage, hypnotic gastric banding is a safe and natural alternative. However, it is important to note that hypnotic gastric band may not be suitable for everyone, and those with underlying medical conditions or severe obesity may require more intensive weight loss interventions.

Evidence of Effectiveness

There have been several studies conducted on the effectiveness of hypnotic gastric band as a weight loss method, with results indicating that it can be an effective alternative to traditional weight loss methods.

A study published in the *International Journal of Clinical and Experimental Hypnosis* in 2014 found that participants who underwent hypnotic gastric banding lost an average of 8.2% of their body weight over a period of six months. Another study published in *the Journal of Consulting and Clinical Psychology* in 2010 found that participants who received hypnotic gastric banding lost an average of 6.8 kg (15 lbs.) over a period of eight weeks.

Success rates for hypnotic gastric band can vary depending on individual factors such as the client's commitment to the program and their overall health and lifestyle habits. However, some studies have reported success rates of up to 75% in terms of achieving significant weight loss.

In comparison to other weight loss methods, hypnotic gastric banding has been found to be more effective than traditional dieting and exercise programs in some cases. For example, a study published in the *American Journal of Clinical Hypnosis* in 2014 found that participants who received hypnotic gastric banding lost significantly more weight than those who received traditional weight loss counseling.

However, it is important to note that hypnotic gastric banding is not a one-size-fits-all solution and may not be suitable for everyone. It is important to consult with a qualified practitioner and to consider other weight loss options before deciding on a course of treatment.

Benefits of Hypnotic Gastric Band

Hypnotic gastric banding is a non-invasive weight loss method that offers several benefits over traditional weight loss surgeries. Here are some of the benefits of hypnotic gastric banding:

Non-invasive and safe:

Hypnotic gastric banding is a safe and non-invasive weight loss method that does not require any surgical incisions or anesthesia. Unlike traditional weight loss surgeries like gastric bypass, gastric sleeve, or Lap-Band, hypnotic gastric banding does not involve cutting or stapling the stomach. This means that there are no risks associated with anesthesia, bleeding, infection, or other complications that can arise from surgery.

No recovery time:

Since hypnotic gastric banding is a non-invasive procedure, there is no recovery time needed. Patients can return to their normal activities immediately after the session. This means that there is no need to take time off work or to arrange for someone to take care of you during the recovery period.

No physical side effects:

Another benefit of hypnotic gastric banding is that there are no physical side effects associated with the procedure. Traditional weight loss surgeries can cause physical discomfort, nausea, vomiting, and other side effects that can last for several weeks or months. With hypnotic gastric banding, there are no physical side effects to worry about.

In addition to these benefits, hypnotic gastric banding is also a cost-effective weight loss method that can be tailored to each individual's needs. It is a safe, non-invasive, and effective way to lose weight and improve your overall health and well-being.

Criticisms of Hypnotic Gastric Band

Hypnotic gastric banding, like any weight loss method, has its share of criticisms. Here are some of the criticisms of hypnotic gastric banding:

Lack of regulation:

Hypnotic gastric banding is not regulated by any governing body, which means that there are no standards or guidelines for the procedure. This lack of regulation can be concerning for some people who may worry about the safety and effectiveness of the procedure.

Skepticism from medical professionals:

Some medical professionals are skeptical about the effectiveness of hypnotic gastric banding. They argue that there is not enough scientific evidence to support the claims made about the procedure. Some also argue that the weight loss achieved through hypnotic gastric banding is not sustainable in the long-term.

Cost:

Like any weight loss method, hypnotic gastric banding can be expensive. Some people may not be able to afford the cost of the procedure, which can be a barrier to accessing this form of treatment.

While hypnotic gastric banding has benefits, it is not without its criticisms. The lack of regulation, skepticism from medical professionals, and cost are some of the criticisms that may make people hesitant to try this weight loss method. It is important to thoroughly research any weight loss method before deciding whether it is right for you.

Who is a Good Candidate for Hypnotic Gastric Band?

Hypnotic gastric banding is a weight loss method that has gained popularity in recent years. It involves using hypnosis to create the sensation of a gastric band in the stomach, which leads to reduced food intake and weight loss. But who is a good candidate for this procedure? Here are some factors that may make a person a good candidate for hypnotic gastric banding:

Individuals who are overweight or obese:

Hypnotic gastric banding is typically recommended for individuals who have a body mass index (BMI) of 30 or above. This is because people who fall into this category are at a higher risk of developing health problems like diabetes, heart disease, and high blood pressure.

Those who have failed with other weight loss methods:

Hypnotic gastric banding may be a good option for people who have tried other weight loss methods, such as diet and exercise, but have not seen significant results. This method may be particularly helpful for people who struggle with emotional eating or have a strong aversion to traditional weight loss methods.

Those who are committed to making lifestyle changes:

Hypnotic gastric banding is not a magic solution for weight loss. It requires a commitment to making lifestyle changes, such as eating a healthy diet and getting regular exercise. People who are committed to making these changes are more likely to see success with hypnotic gastric banding.

People who are overweight or obese, have failed with other weight loss methods, and are committed to making lifestyle changes may be good candidates for hypnotic gastric banding. However, it is important to discuss this option with a healthcare professional to determine if it is the right choice for individual needs and circumstances.

What to Expect During Hypnotic Gastric Band Sessions

If you are considering this method, it is important to know what to expect during the sessions. Here are some factors to consider:

Length of sessions:

Hypnotic gastric banding sessions usually last between 60 and 90 minutes. During this time, the hypnotherapist will guide you into a relaxed state and use visualization techniques to create the sensation of a gastric band in your stomach.

Number of sessions required:

The number of sessions required for hypnotic gastric banding can vary depending on the individual. Some people may see results after just one or two sessions, while others may require several more. Typically, the initial session is followed by several follow-up sessions to reinforce the suggestions made during the initial session.

Cost of sessions:

The cost of hypnotic gastric banding sessions can also vary depending on the practitioner and location. Some practitioners may charge a flat fee for the entire program, while others may charge per session. The cost can range from a few hundred to several thousand dollars.

It is important to note that hypnotic gastric banding is not a magic solution for weight loss. It requires a commitment to making lifestyle changes, such as eating a healthy diet and getting regular exercise. Hypnotic gastric banding should be considered as a supplement to a healthy lifestyle, rather than a replacement for it.

Hypnotic gastric banding sessions typically last between 60 and 90 minutes, the number of sessions required can vary, and the cost can also vary depending on the practitioner and location. It is important to discuss this option with a healthcare professional to determine if it is the right choice for individual needs and circumstances.

Summary

Hypnotic gastric banding has shown to be an effective weight loss method for many individuals. The benefits of this approach include a non-invasive technique that creates the sensation of a gastric band in the stomach without the risks associated with surgery. It is a method that encourages individuals to make positive lifestyle changes by reducing food intake and promoting a healthier diet.

If you are considering hypnotic gastric banding as a weight loss method, it is important to know what to expect during sessions. The length of sessions can range from 60 to 90 minutes, and the number of sessions required can vary based on individual needs. The cost of sessions can also vary depending on the practitioner and location.

We encourage individuals to consider hypnotic gastric banding as a supplement to a healthy lifestyle. It is not a magic solution for weight loss but can be an effective tool for those who are committed to making positive lifestyle changes. It is important to discuss this option with a healthcare professional to determine if it is the right choice for individual needs and circumstances.

In conclusion, if you are looking for a non-invasive weight loss method that can help you make positive lifestyle changes, hypnotic gastric banding may be worth considering. With commitment and dedication, it can be an effective tool for achieving your weight loss goals.

Part IV: The Process of Hypnotic Gastric Band

Unlike traditional gastric band surgery, there are no incisions or physical alterations made to the body during this procedure. However, proper preparation is still necessary to ensure the safety and effectiveness of the treatment. In this part of the book, we will provide an overview of the preparation process for hypnotic gastric banding, including medical evaluation, hypnotherapy sessions, and ongoing support and follow-up.

Medical Evaluation

Medical evaluation is an important step in the process of hypnotic gastric banding. Before undergoing this non-surgical weight loss method, individuals should have a thorough medical examination to ensure they are suitable candidates for the procedure. This evaluation helps to identify any underlying medical conditions that may pose a risk during the hypnotherapy sessions.

During the evaluation, the medical professional will discuss the individual's medical history, including any previous surgeries or health conditions. They may also evaluate the individual's current weight, BMI, and other vital signs to determine their overall health and fitness level. This information is important in identifying any potential risks associated with the procedure.

It is important to note that hypnotic gastric banding is not recommended for individuals with certain medical conditions, such as diabetes, heart disease, or high blood pressure. The medical evaluation will help to identify any potential risks and ensure that the procedure is safe for the individual.

Once the medical evaluation is complete, the individual will meet with a hypnotherapist to begin the procedure. During the hypnotherapy session, the hypnotherapist will guide the individual into a state of relaxation and suggest the sensation of a gastric band in the stomach. This sensation will help the individual to feel fuller faster and reduce their food intake, leading to weight loss over time.

Overall, a thorough medical evaluation is an important aspect of hypnotic gastric banding to ensure the safety and effectiveness of the procedure. By identifying any potential risks and discussing medical history, individuals can feel confident in their decision to pursue this non-surgical weight loss method.

Discussion of Goals and Expectations

Before undergoing hypnotic gastric banding, it is important to have a clear discussion of weight loss goals and expectations. This conversation helps to set realistic expectations and ensure that the individual is committed to making the necessary lifestyle changes to achieve their goals.

The first step in this discussion is to identify the individual's weight loss goals. This includes determining their target weight, the amount of weight they hope to lose, and the timeline for achieving their goals. It is important to set realistic goals that are achievable with the help of the hypnotic gastric banding procedure.

It is also important to emphasize the importance of lifestyle changes and commitment in achieving weight loss goals. While hypnotic gastric banding can be an effective tool for weight loss, it is not a magic solution. Individuals must be committed to making lasting changes to their diet and exercise habits to achieve long-term weight loss success. This includes adopting a healthy, balanced diet and engaging in regular physical activity.

During the discussion of expectations, it is important to be transparent about the potential outcomes of the hypnotic gastric banding procedure. While weight loss is a common outcome, the amount of weight lost and the timeline for achieving weight loss goals can vary from person to person. It is important to communicate that this process may take time and that patience and commitment are key.

Other potential outcomes of the procedure may include changes in eating habits, such as feeling fuller faster and reduced food cravings. Individuals may also experience improved self-confidence and self-esteem as they achieve their weight loss goals.

A discussion of goals and expectations is an important aspect of hypnotic gastric banding to ensure that individuals are committed to making the necessary lifestyle changes and have a realistic understanding of the potential outcomes of the procedure.

Hypnotherapy Sessions

Hypnotherapy sessions are a type of therapy that uses hypnosis to help individuals achieve their goals, overcome obstacles, and improve their overall wellbeing. In the case of hypnotic gastric banding, these sessions are designed to create the sensation of a gastric band without the need for surgery.

The process of creating the sensation of a gastric band involves deep relaxation and visualization techniques. During the session, the hypnotherapist will guide the individual into a state of deep relaxation where they are more receptive to positive suggestions. Once in this state, the hypnotherapist will guide the individual through a visualization exercise where they imagine the sensation of a gastric band being placed around their stomach. This visualization is designed to create a subconscious belief that the individual's stomach is smaller, which can lead to feelings of fullness and reduced appetite.

In addition to the visualization exercise, hypnotherapy sessions often include relaxation techniques and positive affirmations. Relaxation techniques, such as deep breathing and progressive muscle relaxation, are used to help individuals reduce stress and anxiety, which can be a barrier to achieving weight loss goals. Positive affirmations are statements that are repeated to help individuals overcome negative self-talk and develop a positive mindset. These affirmations may focus on self-confidence, motivation, and a belief in the ability to achieve weight loss goals.

Hypnotherapy sessions for hypnotic gastric banding are designed to help individuals create a subconscious belief that their stomach is smaller, which can lead to reduced appetite and weight loss. These sessions often include relaxation techniques and positive affirmations to help individuals develop a positive mindset and overcome obstacles to achieving their weight loss goals. With the guidance of a trained hypnotherapist, individuals can achieve lasting weight loss success through the power of their subconscious mind.

Support and Follow-Up

Support and follow-up are critical components of any weight loss program, including hypnotic gastric banding. The process of losing weight can be challenging, and having a support system in place can help individuals stay motivated and on track. Additionally, regular follow-up appointments are necessary to monitor progress, adjust the program as needed, and address any challenges that may arise.

During the hypnotic gastric banding procedure, it is essential to have a supportive environment. This includes working with a trained hypnotherapist who can guide individuals through the process and provide encouragement and support. Additionally, having a support system of family and friends who are aware of the procedure and can offer encouragement and motivation can be incredibly beneficial.

After the procedure, follow-up appointments are essential to monitor progress and address any issues that may arise. These appointments may include counseling sessions with the hypnotherapist, weigh-ins, and other assessments to track progress. Follow-up appointments can also provide opportunities to adjust the program as needed, such as modifying the visualization exercises or relaxation techniques to better suit the individual's needs.

Despite the many benefits of hypnotic gastric banding, challenges may arise during the weight loss journey. For example, some individuals may struggle with emotional eating or have difficulty sticking to the program. Strategies for overcoming these challenges may include identifying triggers for emotional eating and developing alternative coping mechanisms, such as exercise or meditation. Additionally, working with a counselor or therapist can be helpful for addressing any underlying psychological factors that may be contributing to weight gain.

Support and follow-up are critical components of any weight loss program, including hypnotic gastric banding. Having a supportive environment and regular follow-up appointments can help individuals stay motivated and on track, while also providing opportunities to adjust the program as needed and address any challenges that may arise. With the right support and guidance, individuals can achieve lasting weight loss success through the power of their subconscious mind.

Hypnotic gastric banding is a unique approach to weight loss that focuses on reprogramming the subconscious mind. The preparation process involves careful consideration of one's goals, beliefs, and motivations, as well as working with a trained hypnotherapist to develop a personalized program. This approach can be particularly beneficial for individuals who have struggled with traditional weight loss methods, as it addresses the psychological factors that contribute to weight gain.

It is important to note that hypnotic gastric banding should not be seen as a replacement for a healthy lifestyle. Rather, it should be considered as a supplement to healthy eating habits and regular exercise. By combining hypnotic gastric banding with a healthy lifestyle, individuals can achieve lasting weight loss success and improve their overall health and well-being.

If you are struggling with weight loss, it may be worth considering hypnotic gastric banding as a unique and effective approach. With the right preparation, support, and commitment, this procedure can help you achieve your weight loss goals and improve your quality of life. Remember to always consult with a qualified hypnotherapist and medical professional before pursuing any weight loss program.

CHAPTER 8: THE HYPNOTIC SESSION

The Preparation Process

The preparation process for hypnotic gastric band is a crucial step in achieving success with this weight loss method. It involves several key components, including consultation with a hypnotherapist, assessment of goals and motivations, development of a personalized program, and education about the procedure and expectations.

Consultation with a hypnotherapist:

The first step in the preparation process is to schedule a consultation with a hypnotherapist who specializes in hypnotic gastric band. During this consultation, the hypnotherapist will explain the procedure and answer any questions the patient may have. The hypnotherapist will also assess the patient's suitability for the procedure and determine whether the patient is a good candidate.

Assessment of goals and motivations:

The next step is to assess the patient's goals and motivations for losing weight. The hypnotherapist will ask the patient about their current weight, their weight loss goals, and their reasons for wanting to lose weight. The hypnotherapist will also discuss the patient's eating habits and lifestyle to determine areas where changes can be made.

Development of a personalized program:

Based on the assessment of the patient's goals and motivations, the hypnotherapist will develop a personalized program for the patient. This program will include the number of hypnotic sessions required, the specific suggestions and visualizations that will be used during the sessions, and any additional support that may be needed.

Education about the procedure and expectations:

Finally, the hypnotherapist will educate the patient about the hypnotic gastric band procedure and what to expect during the sessions. The hypnotherapist will also discuss the potential benefits and risks of the procedure and provide guidance on how to maintain a healthy lifestyle after the procedure is completed.

Overall, the preparation process for hypnotic gastric band is an important step in achieving long-term weight loss success. By working with a qualified hypnotherapist, patients can develop a personalized program that is tailored to their individual needs and goals. This program can help patients overcome the psychological barriers that have prevented them from losing weight in the past and achieve lasting results.

The Hypnotic Session

The hypnotic session for hypnotic gastric band is a crucial step in the weight loss process. During the session, the hypnotherapist will use various techniques to help the patient enter a state of trance and visualization. The session will include the following components:

Induction of relaxation and trance:

The first step in the hypnotic session is to induce a state of relaxation and trance. The hypnotherapist will use techniques such as deep breathing, progressive muscle relaxation, and guided imagery to help the patient relax and enter a trance-like state. This state is necessary for the patient to be receptive to the hypnotic suggestions that will be given during the session.

Visualization of the gastric band placement:

Once the patient is in a state of trance, the hypnotherapist will guide them through a visualization exercise. This exercise involves imagining the placement of a gastric band around their stomach. The hypnotherapist will describe the band in detail, including its size, shape, and position. The patient will be encouraged to visualize the band as vividly as possible.

Suggestion of physical sensations and changes:

As the patient visualizes the gastric band placement, the hypnotherapist will suggest physical sensations and changes associated with the procedure. For example, the patient may feel a sense of tightness or fullness in their stomach. The hypnotherapist may also suggest that the patient's appetite is reduced, and they feel satisfied with smaller portions of food.

Reinforcement of healthy eating habits and lifestyle changes:

In addition to the hypnotic suggestions related to the gastric band placement, the hypnotherapist will also reinforce healthy eating habits and lifestyle changes. The patient may be encouraged to eat more slowly, chew their food thoroughly, and make healthier food choices. The hypnotherapist may also suggest that the patient increase their physical activity and incorporate other healthy habits into their daily routine.

Post-hypnotic suggestions for continued success:

Finally, the hypnotherapist will give post-hypnotic suggestions to the patient to reinforce the hypnotic session and promote continued success. These suggestions may include reminders to visualize the gastric band placement regularly, to continue making healthy choices, and to listen to the hypnotic session recording daily.

Overall, the hypnotic session for hypnotic gastric band is a powerful tool for weight loss. By using visualization and suggestion techniques, the hypnotherapist can help the patient overcome psychological barriers to weight loss and achieve long-term success.

Aftercare and Follow-Up

Aftercare and follow-up are essential components of the hypnotic gastric band program. These components ensure that the patient is supported throughout their weight loss journey and can make adjustments as needed. The following are the key aspects of aftercare and follow-up for the hypnotic gastric band program:

Monitoring of progress and adjustments to the program:

After the initial hypnotic session, the hypnotherapist will monitor the patient's progress and make adjustments to the program as needed.

The hypnotherapist may use various tools to monitor progress, such as weight measurements, food diaries, and feedback from the patient. Based on this information, the hypnotherapist can make adjustments to the hypnotic suggestions and provide additional support as needed.

Continued support from the hypnotherapist:

The hypnotic gastric band program requires ongoing support from the hypnotherapist to ensure the patient's success. The hypnotherapist will provide ongoing support through regular follow-up sessions, phone or email support, and access to educational resources. This support can help the patient stay motivated and on track with their weight loss goals.

Recommendations for healthy eating and exercise:

As part of the aftercare and follow-up process, the hypnotherapist will provide recommendations for healthy eating and exercise. These recommendations are based on the patient's individual needs and goals and may include tips for meal planning, portion control, and exercise routines. By following these recommendations, the patient can continue to make progress towards their weight loss goals.

Refresher sessions as needed:

Over time, the hypnotic suggestions may need to be reinforced or adjusted to ensure continued success. The hypnotherapist may recommend refresher sessions as needed to help the patient maintain their progress and stay motivated. These sessions can help the patient overcome any new psychological barriers to weight loss and provide additional support as needed.

Aftercare and follow-up are essential components of the hypnotic gastric band program. By providing ongoing support, recommendations for healthy eating and exercise, and refresher sessions as needed, the hypnotherapist can help the patient achieve long-term success and maintain their weight loss goals.

Summary

The hypnotic gastric band is a non-invasive and effective weight loss procedure that can help individuals achieve their weight loss goals. The process involves a hypnotherapist inducing a trance-like state and suggesting that the patient has undergone a surgical gastric band procedure. This suggestion can help the patient reduce their food intake and lose weight.

While the hypnotic gastric band is generally safe, there are potential risks such as the possibility of not achieving the desired level of weight loss, and the patient's reliance on the hypnotherapist. However, the benefits of the procedure include a non-invasive, pain-free, and cost-effective approach to weight loss.

It is important to note that the hypnotic gastric band is intended to be a supplement to a healthy lifestyle, including healthy eating habits and regular exercise. The procedure can help individuals break through psychological barriers to weight loss and provide additional support to achieve their goals.

The hypnotic gastric band is a viable option for individuals seeking a non-invasive and effective approach to weight loss. We encourage those interested in the procedure to research and consult with a qualified hypnotherapist to determine if it is the right option for them. With the right mindset and support, individuals can achieve their weight loss goals and improve their overall health and wellbeing.

CHAPTER 9: THE POST-HYPNOTIC PERIOD

The Process of Hypnotic Gastric Band

The process of hypnotic gastric band is a weight loss technique that uses hypnotherapy to simulate the effects of gastric band surgery. This non-invasive procedure aims to help people lose weight by changing their mindset and behavior towards food. The process involves several stages, including preparation for hypnosis, induction of hypnosis, and post-hypnotic instructions.

Preparation for Hypnosis:

The first step in the process of hypnotic gastric band is the initial consultation. During this meeting, the hypnotherapist will assess the client's suitability for the procedure and discuss their weight loss goals. The therapist will also explain the process of hypnosis and answer any questions the client may have.

After the consultation, the client will need to mentally prepare themselves for the hypnosis session. This may involve practicing relaxation techniques, such as mindfulness or deep breathing exercises, to help them enter a state of calm and focus.

Induction of Hypnosis:

The induction of hypnosis is the second stage of the process. During this stage, the hypnotherapist will guide the client into a trance-like state using relaxation techniques. The client will be asked to close their eyes and focus on their breathing while the therapist uses calming language to help them relax.

Once the client is in a deep state of relaxation, the therapist will suggest the sensation of undergoing gastric band surgery. The therapist will use visualization techniques to make the client believe that they have undergone the surgery and that their stomach has been reduced in size.

Post-Hypnotic Instructions:

The final stage of the process is the post-hypnotic instructions. During this stage, the hypnotherapist will reinforce the suggestion of the gastric band surgery and encourage the client to make healthy lifestyle changes.

The therapist may suggest changes to the client's diet, such as reducing portion sizes or avoiding certain types of food. The therapist may also encourage the client to exercise regularly and practice stress-reducing techniques like yoga or meditation.

Follow-up sessions are also a crucial part of the process. The hypnotherapist will need to monitor the client's progress and provide ongoing support to help them maintain their weight loss. These sessions may involve further hypnosis or counseling to address any emotional or psychological issues that may be contributing to the client's weight gain.

The process of hypnotic gastric band involves several stages, including preparation for hypnosis, induction of hypnosis, and post-hypnotic instructions. This non-invasive weight loss technique aims to change the client's mindset and behavior towards food and encourage healthy lifestyle changes. Follow-up sessions are essential to help clients maintain their weight loss and address any underlying emotional or psychological issues.

The Post-Hypnotic Period

The post-hypnotic period is a crucial stage in the process of hypnotic gastric band. This is the period after the hypnosis session when the client must adjust to the suggestion of gastric band surgery and make lifestyle changes to maintain their weight loss. The post-hypnotic period can be challenging, but with the right support and guidance, clients can successfully lose weight and keep it off.

Adjustment Period:

The first stage of the post-hypnotic period is the adjustment period. During this stage, clients may experience physical and psychological effects as they adapt to the suggestion of gastric band surgery. Physical effects may include changes in appetite, digestion, and bowel movements. Psychological effects may include changes in mood, self-esteem, and body image.

Maintenance of Weight Loss:

The second stage of the post-hypnotic period is the maintenance of weight loss. During this stage, clients must make lifestyle changes to maintain their weight loss. This may involve making changes to their diet, such as reducing portion sizes, avoiding certain types of food, and eating more fruits and vegetables. It may also involve incorporating regular exercise into their routine and practicing stress-reducing techniques like meditation or yoga.

Continued hypnotherapy can also be beneficial during the maintenance stage. This may involve further hypnosis sessions to reinforce the suggestion of gastric band surgery and address any emotional or psychological issues that may be contributing to the client's weight gain.

Potential Challenges:

The post-hypnotic period can be challenging for clients, and there are several potential challenges that they may face.

1. Temptations and Cravings: Clients may experience temptations and cravings for unhealthy foods, especially during social events or when feeling stressed. It is important to have strategies in place to deal with these cravings, such as finding healthy alternatives or practicing mindfulness.

2. Emotional Triggers: Emotional triggers, such as stress, anxiety, or boredom, may lead to overeating. Clients should work with their hypnotherapist to identify and address these triggers and develop healthy coping mechanisms.

3. Support System: Having a support system, such as family, friends, or a support group, can be beneficial during the post-hypnotic period. Support can provide encouragement, accountability, and motivation.

The post-hypnotic period is a crucial stage in the process of hypnotic gastric band. Clients must adjust to the suggestion of gastric band surgery and make lifestyle changes to maintain their weight loss. Continued hypnotherapy can be beneficial during the maintenance stage, and clients may face challenges such as temptations and cravings, emotional triggers, and the need for a support system. With the right support and guidance, clients can successfully lose weight and keep it off.

Summary

Hypnotic gastric band is a non-invasive and effective weight loss alternative that utilizes the power of suggestion to help clients lose weight. The process of hypnotic gastric band involves a series of hypnosis sessions that suggest the presence of a gastric band in the stomach, leading to reduced appetite and increased satiety.

The post-hypnotic period is a crucial stage in the process of hypnotic gastric band. During this period, clients must adjust to the suggestion of gastric band surgery and make lifestyle changes to maintain their weight loss. The post-hypnotic period may present challenges, such as temptations, emotional triggers, and the need for a support system.

However, with the right support and guidance, clients can successfully lose weight and keep it off. It is important to work with a qualified and experienced hypnotherapist who can tailor the treatment to the client's individual needs and provide ongoing support during the post-hypnotic period.

If you have struggled with weight loss through traditional methods and are considering hypnotic gastric band, we encourage you to explore this option further. Hypnotic gastric band has helped many people achieve their weight loss goals and improve their overall health and well-being.

In summary, we recommend that you consider hypnotic gastric band as a safe and effective weight loss solution. With the right mindset, lifestyle changes, and support, you can achieve long-term weight loss success and improve your quality of life.

CHAPTER 10: FOLLOW-UP CARE AND SUPPORT

Follow-up care and support are essential components of any weight loss program, including hypnotic gastric band. The post-hypnotic period is a critical time for individuals who have undergone hypnotic gastric band treatment, as it is the time when they must make significant lifestyle changes to achieve long-term success.

Importance of the Post-Hypnotic Period:

The post-hypnotic period is the time immediately following the hypnotic gastric band treatment. During this period, individuals must maintain their motivation, work towards their goals, and make lifestyle changes necessary for success. The post-hypnotic suggestions provided by the hypnotherapist help individuals to focus on healthy eating habits, regular exercise, and self-care. Individuals must embrace these changes to ensure long-term success.

Lifestyle Changes Needed for Success:

Lifestyle changes are critical to the success of hypnotic gastric band treatment. These changes include healthy eating habits, regular exercise, and self-care. Individuals must focus on eating a balanced diet, avoiding processed foods, and reducing their calorie intake. Regular exercise is also essential for weight loss and overall health. Self-care practices such as stress reduction, getting enough sleep, and taking time for oneself can also help individuals achieve long-term success.

Emotional and Psychological Support:

Hypnotic gastric band treatment not only addresses the physical aspects of weight loss but also the emotional and psychological aspects. It is essential to address the underlying emotional and psychological factors that contribute to weight gain. Hypnotherapists provide emotional and psychological support to their clients to help them overcome these challenges. Support can include counseling, therapy, and other resources.

Support Groups and Resources:

Support groups and resources can also play a critical role in the success of hypnotic gastric band treatment. These groups provide a safe and supportive environment where individuals can share their experiences and receive encouragement and motivation. Other resources include online support groups, books, and other educational materials.

Follow-up care and support are critical components of hypnotic gastric band treatment. The post-hypnotic period is a critical time for individuals to make the necessary lifestyle changes to achieve long-term success. Emotional and psychological support, along with support groups and resources, can help individuals overcome the challenges they face and achieve their weight loss goals.

Benefits of Follow-up Care and Support

Follow-up care and support are essential components of any weight loss program, including hypnotic gastric band. When individuals receive ongoing support and follow-up care, they can experience a range of benefits that contribute to their long-term success.

Increased Success Rates:

Studies have shown that individuals who receive follow-up care and support after hypnotic gastric band treatment have higher success rates than those who do not. This is because ongoing support helps individuals stay motivated, maintain healthy habits, and overcome any challenges they may face.

Improved Long-Term Weight Loss:

Hypnotic gastric band treatment can lead to significant weight loss in the short term, but maintaining this weight loss over the long term can be challenging. Follow-up care and support can help individuals maintain their weight loss by providing ongoing motivation and accountability. This can lead to improved long-term weight loss and a healthier lifestyle.

Better Overall Health and Well-being:

The benefits of follow-up care and support extend beyond weight loss. Individuals who receive ongoing support after hypnotic gastric band treatment may experience improved overall health and well-being. This can include improved blood sugar control, lower blood pressure, and reduced risk of chronic diseases such as heart disease and diabetes.

Improved Mental Health:

Follow-up care and support can also benefit an individual's mental health. Hypnotic gastric band treatment can be a significant life change, and individuals may experience anxiety, stress, or other emotional challenges. Ongoing support can help individuals manage these challenges and improve their mental health.

Follow-up care and support are essential components of hypnotic gastric band treatment. The benefits of ongoing support include increased success rates, improved long-term weight loss, better overall health and well-being, and improved mental health. Individuals who receive ongoing support after hypnotic gastric band treatment are more likely to achieve their weight loss goals and maintain a healthy lifestyle over the long term.

Summary

Hypnotic gastric band treatment is a viable weight loss option that involves using the power of the mind to create a sense of fullness and reduce food intake. The treatment process involves several sessions, during which a trained hypnotherapist will guide the individual through the process of visualizing a gastric band being placed around their stomach. While hypnotic gastric band treatment can be effective in the short term, it is important to note that maintaining long-term weight loss requires ongoing support and follow-up care. This support can come in many forms, including regular check-ins with a hypnotherapist, support groups, and online resources. It is important to seek out these resources to ensure that you have the best chance of success on your weight loss journey. With the right support and tools, you can achieve your weight loss goals and improve your overall health and well-being.

Part V: Advantages and Disadvantages of Hypnotic Gastric Band

This technique has several advantages over traditional weight loss surgeries, such as no surgery needed, no physical discomfort or pain, no risks or complications associated with surgery, and cost-effectiveness. However, like any other weight loss method, Hypnotic Gastric Band also has some disadvantages that need to be considered. In this part of the book, we will discuss both the advantages and disadvantages of Hypnotic Gastric Band.

CHAPTER 11: ADVANTAGES

Hypnotic Gastric Band has several advantages over traditional weight loss surgeries. It is non-invasive, painless, free of complications, requires no recovery time, leaves no scars, and is cost-effective. These benefits make it an attractive option for those who are looking to lose weight without the risks and expenses associated with surgery.

Hypnotic Gastric Band is a non-invasive weight loss procedure that has several advantages over traditional weight loss surgeries. In addition to the benefits mentioned in the previous section, Hypnotic Gastric Band also offers the following advantages:

No recovery time required: Unlike traditional weight loss surgeries, patients who undergo Hypnotic Gastric Band do not require any recovery time. This means that they can resume their daily activities immediately after the procedure, without any restrictions.

No scars or marks left on the body: Weight loss surgeries, such as gastric bypass or sleeve gastrectomy, require incisions that leave scars or marks on the body. In contrast, Hypnotic Gastric Band is a non-invasive procedure that does not leave any scars or marks on the body. This is particularly beneficial for those who are concerned about cosmetic issues associated with weight loss surgeries.

Cost-effective compared to surgery: Weight loss surgeries can be expensive, with costs ranging from thousands to tens of thousands of dollars. Hypnotic Gastric Band, on the other hand, is much more affordable, making it accessible to a wider range of people. This cost-effectiveness is a significant advantage for those who cannot afford the high costs of traditional weight loss surgeries.

Hypnotic Gastric Band is a non-invasive weight loss procedure that has several advantages over traditional weight loss surgeries. Its benefits include no recovery time required, no scars or marks left on the body, and cost-effectiveness compared to surgery. These advantages make Hypnotic Gastric Band an attractive option for those seeking a safe, affordable, and effective weight loss solution.

Psychological Benefits

Addresses emotional and psychological triggers of overeating:

Hypnotic Gastric Band helps individuals to identify and address the emotional and psychological triggers of overeating. This technique involves reprogramming the subconscious mind to change negative thought patterns and behaviors that contribute to overeating.

Helps to change unhealthy eating habits:

Hypnotic Gastric Band helps individuals to develop healthy eating habits and behaviors. This technique encourages individuals to listen to their bodies, eat mindfully, and make healthier food choices. By doing so, individuals can develop a healthier relationship with food, which can lead to long-term weight loss success.

Boosts self-confidence and improves body image:

Hypnotic Gastric Band can help individuals to feel more confident and positive about their bodies. This technique encourages individuals to focus on their strengths and accomplishments rather than their perceived flaws. As a result, individuals can develop a more positive body image and improve their self-confidence.

Promotes a healthier lifestyle:

Hypnotic Gastric Band promotes a healthier lifestyle by encouraging individuals to adopt healthy habits, such as regular exercise and stress management. This technique helps individuals to make positive changes in their lives, which can lead to improved health and well-being.

In conclusion, Hypnotic Gastric Band offers several psychological benefits, including addressing emotional and psychological triggers of overeating, helping to change unhealthy eating habits, boosting self-confidence and improving body image, and promoting a healthier lifestyle. These psychological benefits can have a significant impact on an individual's overall health and well-being, making Hypnotic Gastric Band a valuable tool for weight loss and psychological wellness.

Long-term Benefits

Sustainable weight loss:

Hypnotic Gastric Band helps individuals to achieve sustainable weight loss by promoting healthy lifestyle habits such as regular exercise and a balanced diet. These habits help individuals maintain their weight loss over the long term, rather than experiencing temporary weight loss that is regained after a short period.

Maintains weight loss for a longer period:

Hypnotic Gastric Band helps individuals maintain their weight loss for a longer period of time. Unlike other weight loss methods, such as crash diets or weight loss pills that offer temporary results, Hypnotic Gastric Band helps individuals change their relationship with food and develop healthier habits that can be maintained over the long term.

Improves overall health and reduces the risk of obesity-related diseases:

Hypnotic Gastric Band not only helps individuals lose weight but also improves their overall health. Being overweight or obese can increase the risk of several health problems such as diabetes, high blood pressure, heart disease, and stroke. By achieving sustainable weight loss, individuals can reduce their risk of these diseases and improve their overall health.

Hypnotic Gastric Band offers several long-term benefits, including sustainable weight loss, maintaining weight loss for a longer period, and improving overall health. These benefits make Hypnotic Gastric Band a valuable tool for individuals who are struggling with obesity and are looking for a safe and effective weight loss method that can improve their overall health and well-being.

Summary

Hypnotic Gastric Band helps individuals address emotional and psychological triggers of overeating, change unhealthy eating habits, boost self-confidence and improve body image, promote a healthier lifestyle, achieve sustainable weight loss, maintain weight loss for a longer period, and improve overall health while reducing the risk of obesity-related diseases.

If you are struggling with obesity and are looking for a safe and effective weight loss method, Hypnotic Gastric Band is an option worth considering. With its long-term benefits and psychological advantages, it can help you achieve your weight loss goals while improving your overall health and well-being.

CHAPTER 12: DISADVANTAGES

While this method offers several benefits such as sustainable weight loss and psychological advantages, it is important to acknowledge that it also has some disadvantages that need to be considered. Before deciding whether to undergo Hypnotic Gastric Band, it is important to understand its potential drawbacks and how they may affect individual circumstances. This chapter will explore the disadvantages of Hypnotic Gastric Band and provide insights into how to make an informed decision.

Disadvantages of Hypnotic Gastric Band

Limited effectiveness:

While Hypnotic Gastric Band has been shown to be effective for some individuals, it is not suitable for everyone. People who have underlying medical conditions, such as gastrointestinal disorders or mental health issues, may not be good candidates for this method. Additionally, the effectiveness of Hypnotic Gastric Band can vary from person to person. Some individuals may experience significant weight loss, while others may not see much difference in their weight.

Cost:

The cost of Hypnotic Gastric Band can be a significant disadvantage for some people. Hypnotherapy sessions can be expensive, and multiple sessions may be required to achieve the desired results. In addition to the cost of the hypnotherapy sessions, there may be additional expenses for follow-up sessions or dietary supplements recommended by the practitioner. This can make Hypnotic Gastric Band a costly weight loss option, particularly for those on a tight budget.

Time-consuming:

Another disadvantage of Hypnotic Gastric Band is that it can be time-consuming. Multiple hypnotherapy sessions may be required to achieve the desired results, and each session can take several hours. Additionally, achieving sustainable weight loss through Hypnotic Gastric Band requires a commitment to making lifestyle changes. This can be time-consuming and may require significant effort and dedication.

Time-consuming:

Hypnotic Gastric Band is a time-consuming weight loss option that requires multiple hypnotherapy sessions. Each session can take several hours, and several sessions may be required to achieve the desired results. Additionally, achieving sustainable weight loss through Hypnotic Gastric Band requires a commitment to making lifestyle changes, which can also be time-consuming. This can make Hypnotic Gastric Band a challenging weight loss option for individuals with busy schedules or those who have difficulty making time for self-care.

Psychological challenges:

While Hypnotic Gastric Band can be effective for some individuals, it may not be suitable for those with underlying psychological issues. Hypnotherapy relies on the power of suggestion to change behavior, and individuals with certain psychological conditions, such as anxiety or depression, may not respond well to this approach. Additionally, Hypnotic Gastric Band can lead to frustration, disappointment, and relapse for some individuals who do not see the desired results. This can have negative psychological effects and may make it difficult to maintain healthy habits over the long term.

While Hypnotic Gastric Band offers some benefits for weight loss, it is important to consider the potential disadvantages before deciding to undergo this approach. Time commitment, psychological challenges, and limited effectiveness are some of the factors to consider when evaluating whether Hypnotic Gastric Band is the right weight loss option for an individual. It is important to consult with a healthcare professional before making any decisions about weight loss methods and to prioritize overall health and well-being.

Summary

Hypnotic Gastric Band is a weight loss option that offers some potential benefits, such as sustainable weight loss. However, it also has several disadvantages that should be carefully considered before deciding to undergo this method. These disadvantages include limited effectiveness, cost, time commitment, and psychological challenges. It is important to acknowledge that the effectiveness of Hypnotic Gastric Band can vary from person to person and that certain individuals may not be good candidates for this approach due to underlying medical or psychological conditions.

Therefore, before making a decision, it is important to consider individual circumstances and consult with a healthcare professional. A healthcare professional can provide guidance and support to help determine the best weight loss method based on an individual's unique needs and preferences. Ultimately, the most important consideration should be overall health and well-being, and any weight loss approach should be implemented in conjunction with a balanced diet, regular exercise, and healthy lifestyle habits.

CHAPTER 13: COMPARISON WITH OTHER WEIGHT LOSS METHODS

In today's world, obesity has become a major health concern. It is associated with various health problems, including heart disease, diabetes, and high blood pressure. As a result, there has been an increasing demand for weight loss methods. One such method is the hypnotic gastric band, a technique that uses hypnosis to simulate the effects of gastric band surgery. While this approach has gained popularity in recent years, it is important to compare it with other weight loss methods to determine its effectiveness, cost, time commitment, and potential risks and side effects when compared to other treatments. This comparison will help individuals make an informed decision about which weight loss method will be most effective for their unique needs and circumstances. In this chapter, we will compare hypnotic gastric band with other weight loss methods to help determine its place in the spectrum of available weight loss treatments.

Other Weight Loss Methods

There are several weight loss methods available in addition to hypnotic gastric band. These methods can be broadly classified into three categories: diet and exercise, medications, and surgery. Each method has its own advantages and disadvantages, which we will discuss in detail below.

1. Diet and Exercise:

Diet and exercise are the most common methods for weight loss. They involve making changes to your diet and increasing physical activity levels. Diet and exercise can be further broken down into several subcategories, such as low-carb diets, high-protein diets, and low-fat diets. Similarly, exercise can include cardio, strength training, and high-intensity interval training (HIIT).

Advantages:

- Diet and exercise are generally safe and effective for weight loss.

- They can also improve overall health and reduce the risk of chronic diseases.

Disadvantages:

- Diet and exercise require a significant commitment of time and effort.

- Results may take longer to achieve than other methods.

2. Medications:

Medications are another option for weight loss. They work by reducing appetite, increasing feelings of fullness, or preventing the absorption of fat.

Advantages:

- Medications can be effective for weight loss, particularly when combined with diet and exercise.

- They can be helpful for individuals who have struggled to lose weight through other methods.

Disadvantages:

- Medications can have potential side effects, and may not be suitable for everyone.

- They may also be expensive and require ongoing use.

3. Surgery:

Surgery is typically considered a last resort for weight loss, and is typically reserved for individuals with a body mass index (BMI) of 40 or higher. There are several types of weight loss surgery, including gastric bypass, gastric sleeve, and adjustable gastric banding.

Advantages:

- Surgery can lead to significant weight loss and may improve overall health.

- It can also be helpful for individuals who have struggled to lose weight through other methods.

Disadvantages:

- Surgery is a major procedure that carries risks and potential complications.

- It can also be expensive and require significant lifestyle changes.

Overall, there are many different weight loss methods available, each with its own set of advantages and disadvantages. It is important to consider individual circumstances and consult with a healthcare professional to determine which method is right for you.

Comparison of Hypnotic Gastric Band with Other Weight Loss Methods

When considering weight loss methods, it is important to compare the effectiveness, cost, time commitment, and potential risks and side effects of each option. Here is a side-by-side comparison of hypnotic gastric band and other weight loss methods:

1. Diet and Exercise:

Effectiveness: Diet and exercise can be effective for weight loss, particularly when combined. However, results may take longer to achieve than other methods.

Cost: The cost of diet and exercise will vary depending on individual preferences and needs, but can be relatively low.

Time commitment: Diet and exercise require a significant commitment of time and effort.

Risks and side effects: Generally safe, but there is a risk of injury with exercise.

2. Medications:

Effectiveness: Medications can be effective for weight loss, particularly when combined with diet and exercise.

Cost: Medications can be expensive and require ongoing use.

Time commitment: Medications require ongoing use. Risks and side effects: Medications can have potential side effects, and may not be suitable for everyone.

3. Surgery:

Effectiveness: Surgery can lead to significant weight loss and may improve overall health.

Cost: Surgery can be expensive and may not be covered by insurance.

Time commitment: Surgery requires a significant time commitment and lifestyle changes.

Risks and side effects: Surgery is a major procedure that carries risks and potential complications.

4. Hypnotic Gastric Band:

Effectiveness: The effectiveness of hypnotic gastric band is still being studied, but early research suggests it may be effective for some individuals.

Cost: The cost of hypnotic gastric band can vary, but it is generally less expensive than surgery.

Time commitment: Hypnotic gastric band requires a significant time commitment, but less than surgery.

Risks and side effects: Hypnotic gastric band is generally considered safe, but there may be some psychological risks associated with hypnosis.

Overall, each weight loss method has its own advantages and disadvantages. It is important to consider individual circumstances and consult with a healthcare professional to determine which method is right for you. While hypnotic gastric band may be a less invasive and less expensive option than surgery, it is important to note that its effectiveness is still being studied and long-term results are not yet known.

Factors to Consider in Choosing a Weight Loss Method

Choosing the right weight loss method can be challenging, as there are many options available and each method has its own advantages and disadvantages. When considering which weight loss method to choose, it is important to take into account individual circumstances and consult with a healthcare professional. Here are some factors to consider when choosing a weight loss method:

1. Health status: It is important to consider any pre-existing health conditions, such as diabetes or heart disease, when choosing a weight loss method. Some methods may be more appropriate for individuals with certain health conditions than others.

2. Weight loss goals: Different weight loss methods may be more effective for different weight loss goals. For example, surgery may be more effective for individuals with a larger amount of weight to lose, while diet and exercise may be more appropriate for individuals with a smaller amount of weight to lose.

3. Lifestyle: It is important to consider lifestyle factors, such as work schedule and family responsibilities, when choosing a weight loss method. Some methods may require more time and effort than others, and may be difficult to incorporate into a busy lifestyle.

4. Budget: The cost of different weight loss methods can vary widely, and it is important to consider the financial impact of each option. Some methods may be covered by insurance, while others may require out-of-pocket expenses.

5. Risks and side effects: It is important to consider the potential risks and side effects of each weight loss method. Some methods may carry more risks than others, and it is important to weigh the potential benefits against the potential risks.

Ultimately, the choice of weight loss method should be tailored to individual circumstances and goals. Consulting with a healthcare professional can help ensure that the most appropriate method is chosen, and that the weight loss journey is undertaken safely and effectively.

Summary

There are several weight loss methods available, each with its own set of advantages and disadvantages. Diet and exercise, medications, surgery, and hypnotic gastric band are all options that can help individuals achieve their weight loss goals. When making a decision, it is important to consider individual circumstances, such as health status, weight loss goals, lifestyle, budget, and potential risks and side effects. The consultation with a healthcare professional is also crucial in determining the most appropriate method for each individual. Although hypnotic gastric band may be a less invasive and less expensive option than surgery, its effectiveness is still being studied, and long-term results are not yet known. Therefore, taking the time to weigh the pros and cons of each method and seeking professional guidance can help ensure that the chosen method is safe, effective, and appropriate for individual needs.

Part VI: Frequently Asked Questions about Hypnotic Gastric Band

Many people may have questions and concerns about the procedure. It is important to address these common questions and concerns to ensure that individuals are making informed decisions about their health and well-being. In this part of the book, we will explore some of the most frequently asked questions about hypnotic gastric band, and provide expert answers and explanations to help individuals make informed decisions about whether this procedure is right for them.

CHAPTER 14: COMMON QUESTIONS AND CONCERNS

Is Hypnotic Gastric Band Safe?

One of the most common concerns about hypnotic gastric band is whether it is safe. Unlike traditional gastric band surgery, which involves physically fitting a band around the stomach, hypnotic gastric band is a non-invasive procedure that uses hypnosis to create the sensation of a band being fitted. While there are some risks associated with any medical procedure, hypnotic gastric band is generally considered to be a safe and low-risk option for weight loss.

How Effective is Hypnotic Gastric Band?

Another common question about hypnotic gastric band is how effective it is at promoting weight loss. The research on hypnotic gastric band is somewhat limited, but there is some evidence to suggest that it can be an effective tool for weight loss. Some studies have found that individuals who undergo hypnotic gastric band lose a significant amount of weight in the short-term, although the long-term effectiveness of the procedure is less clear.

Are There Any Side Effects or Risks?

As with any medical procedure, there are some risks associated with hypnotic gastric band. Common side effects include nausea, vomiting, and dizziness. More serious risks, such as internal bleeding or infection, are rare but can occur. It is important to discuss the potential risks and side effects of hypnotic gastric band with a qualified healthcare professional before undergoing the procedure.

What is the Cost of Hypnotic Gastric Band?

The cost of hypnotic gastric band can vary depending on a number of factors, including the location of the clinic, the qualifications of the practitioner, and the specific details of the procedure. In general, however, hypnotic gastric band is less expensive than traditional gastric band surgery, which can cost tens of thousands of dollars. Some insurance plans may cover the cost of hypnotic gastric band, although this varies depending on the individual plan and the specific procedure being performed.

Can Hypnotic Gastric Band Be Used as a Replacement for Traditional Gastric Band Surgery?

While hypnotic gastric band is a non-invasive alternative to traditional gastric band surgery, it is not typically used as a replacement for the surgical procedure. Traditional gastric band surgery involves physically fitting a band around the stomach to restrict the amount of food that can be consumed. Hypnotic gastric band, on the other hand, uses hypnosis to create the sensation of a band being fitted, without any physical changes to the body. While hypnotic gastric band may be effective for some individuals, it is not considered to be a substitute for traditional gastric band surgery.

Is Hypnotic Gastric Band Covered by Insurance?

The coverage of hypnotic gastric band by insurance varies depending on the individual insurance plan and the specific details of the procedure. While some insurance plans may cover the cost of hypnotic gastric band, others may not. It is important to check with your insurance provider to determine whether hypnotic gastric band is covered under your plan. Additionally, it may be necessary to obtain pre-approval from the insurance company before undergoing the procedure.

Summary

Common questions about hypnotic gastric band include concerns about its safety, effectiveness, side effects and risks, as well as the cost and whether it can replace traditional gastric band surgery. Expert answers indicate that hypnotic gastric band is generally considered safe and effective for weight loss, although it is not typically used as a replacement for traditional surgery. Common side effects include nausea, vomiting, and dizziness. The cost of hypnotic gastric band varies depending on several factors and may or may not be covered by insurance.

It is important to seek professional guidance when considering hypnotic gastric band or any weight loss procedure. A qualified healthcare professional can help determine if hypnotic gastric band is a suitable option for your individual needs and provide guidance on potential risks and side effects. Additionally, a healthcare professional can recommend other weight loss options and provide support throughout the weight loss journey.

While hypnotic gastric band may be a viable weight loss option for some individuals, it is important to carefully consider all options and seek guidance from a qualified healthcare professional before undergoing any weight loss procedure. A holistic approach to weight loss, including a healthy diet and regular exercise, is recommended for long-term success.

Part VII: Final Thoughts

Hypnotic Gastric Banding is a non-surgical weight loss technique that uses hypnosis to simulate the effects of a surgical gastric band. It is a safe and effective option for those looking to lose weight without undergoing surgery, but it is important to make lifestyle changes to support long-term success.

Through expert answers and explanations, it has been shown that Hypnotic Gastric Banding can be an effective way to address hunger and cravings. However, it is important to work with a qualified hypnotherapist and healthcare provider to determine if this technique is right for you.

In terms of future developments, there is ongoing research and advancements in the field of hypnosis and weight loss. As more studies are conducted, we may see further developments in the use of Hypnotic Gastric Banding and other hypnosis-based weight loss techniques.

In conclusion, Hypnotic Gastric Banding is a viable option for those seeking a safe and effective weight loss technique. With the guidance of a qualified hypnotherapist and healthcare provider, it is possible to achieve sustainable weight loss and improve overall health and well-being.

www.ingramcontent.com/pod-product-compliance
Lightning Source LLC
Chambersburg PA
CBHW021337160726

47994CB00007B/2732